I0424036

BODY FORGIVENESS

Weight Loss Testimony

AUDRA M. JOHNSON

~Dedicated to my amazing family and my Son's Father Robert Johnson who lost his battle with obesity in 2009 and those that struggle with Obesity.~

~CONTENTS~

~INTRODUCTION~

WHY THE TITLE BODY FORGIVENESS?

Why the title "Body Forgiveness?" I chose this title because I believe that our body possesses the divine innate ability to forgive itself when we make the changes that are necessary. I'm a living witness and this book is a testimony of how forgiving my body has been to itself.

I have been told by many women over the years how my weight loss success has inspired them. Several of those women have taken the steps necessary to lose weight and live healthier lives. I am now compelled to share my testimony with the world.

My prayer is that this book will motivate, inspire, encourage, bless, everyone that reads it to take action by dealing with unresolved emotional issues and taking control of their health and

wellness.

~*Part One*~

MY CHILDHOOD

JOURNEY

~MY CHILDHOOD STORY~

From childhood and early adolescence, I was an extremely top-heavy "thick girl". I grew up in a two parent household with one sibling. We lived in an upper-middle class neighborhood that was and still is very diverse in culturally.

I began battling the "bulge" at around age ten. People would make comments saying that I ate too much, was fat and that needed to lose weight. Unfortunately, no one ever helped, educated or encouraged me on how to lose weight beyond the negative comments. This left me to my own devices. I thought the only way to lose weight was by not eating or barely eating. I would go on a diet and get on the scale almost every hour hoping and praying that it was going to move. I would rarely exercise as I wasn't a fan of it. The only physical activity I would participate in was short or long distance walking. I even remember how I would compete with a childhood friend to see who could go the longest without eating during the day. I was totally uneducated and doing damage to my metabolism. I even went as far to see how much it would cost to have my mouth wired when I was a teenager.

~MY ELEMENTARY SCHOOL EXPERIENCE~

For me, it all started in Elementary School. I was wearing a training bra by at second grade (I think). Some young girls don't start wearing them until 5th grade and that's at the earliest. Boys at school would chase and tease me on the school yard during recess and lunch. Some would sneak up to me, touch my breasts and run. I would run after them but could never catch them. I would report it to the school yard supervisors and they wouldn't do anything. In today's day and time the way I was treated would be considered a form of child-on-child abuse. I never told my parents because of fear that they would make a large issue of it causing feelings of post-embarrassment.

I believe that's when I began to develop a "shame-driven" complex. I was so ashamed of how my body looked. This went on for many, many, years. By age twelve, I was so top heavy that I began having trouble finding appropriate upper body clothing. It was truly a chore and frustrating for both my mother and I. My bra cup size was a 40D by the time I turned 14 years old.

~MY MIDDLE SCHOOL EXPERIENCE~

Adolescence and Puberty didn't make things better. By the 7th grade I suffered with severe acne, oily skin and severe menstrual cycles. My self-esteem was so low that I experienced a downward spiral that later affected my P.E. (physical education) grades.

I rarely dressed for gym during those years. I didn't like changing clothes in a community dressing room and unfortunately, my grades in that subject suffered because of it. I also had low marks in participation because I would avoid physical activities that involved jumping or running. I remember the mandatory one mile run that was required two times a year. I would start out trying my best but my arches would begin to have a burning sensation that caused me to stop running and start walking. I would always come in close to last. I found that to be very discouraging and would internalize the feelings of failure and defeat thinking something was wrong with me. I realized much later in life that I was wearing improper shoes.

Yes, those middle school years were probably the worst years in my educational experience. I became an introvert personality. So much that I missed my ninth grade pin and ribbon ceremony. My mother was upset after later learning about it months later.

I was excited about my ninth grade graduation ceremony though. I remember how hard it was trying to find a dress that would fit my upper body. Thank God a friend of mine's mother knew a woman that sold clothes. She had something that fit me. Back in those days, stores did not cater to plus size women to the level that they do today.

~MY HIGH SCHOOL EXPERIENCE~

High school wasn't much different. There was much less teasing and ridicule but it was still difficult finding clothes. There were many periods when I would go through sadness because I couldn't wear the "tube tops" "strapless" and "spaghetti strap dresses" and tops like the smaller girls. By this time, I was getting my bras custom made in Beverly Hills, CA. In the early 1980's those bras cost $100.00 each. At that time my parents could only afford to purchase one at a time. That was the only store that I knew of in Los Angeles that could service me.

~MY HIGH SCHOOL PROM~

My High School Prom was what I really looked forward to! I had to have my Prom Dress custom made by a Seamstress. I will never forget how challenging it was to find one because I needed a seamstress that could work without a pattern. There were no patterns around for my size back then. For fittings I would catch 3 public busses and walk about half of a mile one way just to get to the seamstress house in So. Central LA.

She was a really nice plus-sized (size 28-30) married woman. I remember distinctly how sweet and nice she and her entire family were. I thought, finally, I get to wear a spaghetti strap dress. Well, let's say closer to cap sleeves because she insisted that I needed them to support my bust-line. I was really disappointed but lived with it. I had to have a strapless "longline" bra specially made for the dress. My parents paid $150.00 for it! Yes, in 1985, $150.00 U.S. dollars! That was more than the seamstress charged for her labor for sewing the dress! There were times when I would feel so bad about how much money my parents had to pay for my undergarments.

~*Part Two*~

WELCOME TO

ADULTHOOD

~LET THE WEDDINGS BEGIN~

A couple of years after I graduated High School, my sister-friends and high school classmates started getting married. Many of the dresses were spaghetti straps but unfortunately, mine were more like lasagna straps. Each dress was custom made and as usual, I always felt like the "oddball bridesmaid" because my dress was always the "largest" in size amongst all the others. This is when I began researching the possibility of having a breast-reduction.

~THE BREAST REDUCTION~

Finally, I got tired of the bra straps digging into my shoulders, numbness and lower-back pain. At about age 19, I began researching the possibility of having a breast reduction. I learned that my medical insurance coverage would pay the costs to

22

have it done if the required guidelines and qualifications were met.

I later made an appointment with a surgeon for a consultation and discussed the possibility of surgery. During the consultation, I asked the surgeon if I could see photographs of the procedure. He handed me the surgical textbook and turned to the pages that had the photos. I was like, WOW! These were actual photos of the actual surgical procedure! You could see EVERYTHING! After looking at the photos of the actual incisions, I became scared and immediately changed my mind. The surgeon said, ok, you'll be back.

Well the surgeon was right. About six years later, I did return to have breast reduction surgery. The main reason I returned was because the store where I purchased my bra's from closed down and moved to Las Vegas, Nevada. There was no other store that I knew of in LA that made those bras. By the time the store closed I was a size 52FFF.

After a series of consultations and appointments over a period of 6 months, I was scheduled and had the breast reduction surgery. I was 24 years of age. It was a success but the recovery was painful at first. I had layers of consumable stitches on the inside and classic stitches on the outside. The Surgeon wanted me to return for a second surgery to "fine tune" the surgical work. However I elected to pass on the second surgery. I did not want to endure another recovery process and the pain from stitches after post-surgery.

Please don't allow my description to scare you. Today, surgeries of this nature are not as complex. **PLEASE NOTE: I did not have breast-**

reduction surgery to lose weight. I had it to

alleviate years of back pain.

~*Part 3*~

THE TRUTH ABOUT

OBESITY

~LET'S DISCUSS A FEW SIDE AFFECTS OF OBESITY~

My personal belief is that many but not all women that are overweight or obese struggle with maintaining a high level of self-esteem. This can be for a number of different reasons ranging from abuse to T.V. and magazine self comparisons.

Society, acceptance and being ridiculed along with the cruelties in the world associated with being overweight can be overwhelming and take an emotional toll on a woman over time.

~LET'S TALK ABOUT THE DANGERS OF OBESITY~

Obesity in women can lead to many health problems such as High Blood Pressure, Diabetes, Depression, Asthma, Bone, Joint stress and cause a domino effect of other diseases in other areas of health and wellness.

I was well over 300+ pounds at my highest weight with a 5'2 frame. Although I never suffered from the MAJOR diseases like High Blood Pressure and Diabetes, that was way too much weight for me to carry. I did experience foot pain, difficulty breathing on occasion, and lack of energy, sluggishness, a weakened immune system and low self-esteem.

~THE WAKE UP CALL THAT CHANGED MY LIFE~

My wake-up-call was during an annual physical. I was about 38 years of age. During the physical, the Doctor stated to me almost ten times during that visit that I needed to lose weight. I was approaching the age of 40 and he warned me of continuing on that path would make me prone to certain diseases due to obesity and it sunk in. I

finally took it to heart and started my journey a few

weeks later.

~Part 4~

THE PROCESS

~GETTING STARTED~

Usually, the most challenging thing about weight loss is getting started; but once finally take the first step, each day should become less and less challenging.

I got started a few weeks after that Doctor's appointment.

I had just ended an abusive marriage and was going through Divorce #2. I had once again gained an excessive amount of weight during the second marriage because of emotional eating and poor stress management.

I moved out of what was once my dream home into an apartment complex. The complex had a gym on the premises that was only a few yards away from my apartment.

One day, I decided that I would go to the gym.

The first machine I used was the treadmill. I got on the treadmill and began walking with my hands on the handrails. I gained momentum after about 10 minutes and decided to let go of the handrails. My left foot lost traction and I fell down and scarred my knee. I was so embarrassed because other people witnessed me fall!

I immediately picked myself up along with my pride and left the gym. My workout was a total of about 20 minutes. I said to myself that I was not going back there anymore. However, there was something on the inside that wouldn't let me give up so easily. I returned back to the gym the next day. One day led to another I never stopped.

I went from a size 20 to a size 6-8 in about 14 months!

.

~A WOMAN'S ISSUES ARE IN HER BELLY~

Growing up I used hear the older women say, "Honey, a woman's issues are in her belly." I used to think and ask, what does that mean? They would say, just keep on living, you'll know exactly what it means. Well, this is just my opinion but; I believe that it can mean two things. The first thing I believe it means is that women are emotion-driven and have a tendency to reach for comfort foods to sooth and satisfy their emotions and during stressful situations.

Unresolved issues such as unforgiveness, anger, rejection, spiritual entanglements (a.k.a. soul ties) or any other unhealthy emotion can take up unnecessary space causing it to be difficult to lose weight. I know this first hand because I used to major in holding grudges in my younger years. It wasn't until I learned how to let go and release those that hurt me by praying for them and giving my issues to God that I began to see long-term results in my weight loss.

The second are the physical affects. Studies have said that when a woman is under high levels of stress that a hormone called "Cortisol" becomes released. One of the side effects of this hormone is "weight gain" in a woman's abdomen, (belly).

Unresolved emotional issues can later manifest into physical illness.

~TRUE HEALTH AND WELLNESS~

True health and wellness is not just maintaining a healthy weight and proper diet. Total health and wellness involves taking action and control of your total health of the **mind, body,** and **spirit**. It's a lifestyle change that requires the renewing of the mind and consistency in order to be successful. All three must be fed in order to maximize total health and wellness. I feed my mind the Word of God, my body food and my Spirit with Prayer, Affirmations, Decrees, and Meditation.

The key to maintaining all 3 successfully is:
WORK, LIFE AND FAMILY BALANCE.
Balance simply means to position, evenly distribute the weight or enable something or someone to remain upright and steady. It is something that we all must work at and reinforce constantly. It requires evaluating, prioritizing and the 3 R's: Re-Evaluate, Re-Position and Re-Engage.

1. Re-Evaluate involves self-examination and evaluation of the family.
2. Re-Position involves making the necessary changes and developing an action plan.

3. Re-Engage involves putting those necessary changes and new habits to action.

For example, positive confessions or positive affirmations are great ways to train your mind, body and spirit. Exercise or any other physical activity that enhances health and meditation on bible scriptures or pictures feed and enhance the spirit and soul.

~WEIGHT-LOSS~

When it comes to weight loss, results will vary with each individual, their body metabolism, schedule, family dynamics, responsibilities and lifestyle. Never compare your own personal journey with another. Each one of us is different inside and out.

~BELIEVE YOU CAN ACHIEVE IT~

One of the best ways to begin this journey in health, wellness, and weight loss is to begin with the "end in mind". Anything that we accomplish in life will always first begin in your spirit and your mind. Use your imagination and see yourself where you want to be. Make slow gradual changes with consistency and over time and you will see results.

~FIND YOUR "WHY" AND KEEP IT "NEARBY"~

Having a "why" is very important. This form of motivation is one of the things that I used to "jump start" my lifestyle change over eight years ago. It still motivates me to this day. My "why's" are:

- **To live the best quality of life possible for myself and my family**

- **Avoid sicknesses and diseases**

Your "why's" may change periodically and

that's okay but I strongly suggest that you decide on

your "why's" and keep them "nearby".

**Take a moment and write your "why's" below
and reflect on them daily.**

My "Why's":

_____

_____

_____

_____

~*Part 5*~

THE JOURNEY

~CLEANSE (DETOXIFY) YOUR BODY~

Consider detoxifying (cleansing) your body and system at the beginning of your journey. Much of the foods we eat has or is exposed to chemicals and preservatives that can remain in our system. This is especially true when it comes to processed foods. Chemicals and excess food not released from the body over time can attach itself to the colon, kidney, liver and spleen. This is also known as "sludge" in the system. Over time this can cause sickness and disease in the body.

Below is an Olive Oil Cleanse that I do 2 to 3 times each year. Consult with your physician before starting this or any other cleanse regimen.

Olive Oil Cleanse

Purchase a 16oz. bottle of "Cold Pressed" Olive Oil from any health food store.

Drink 8 oz. if you weigh 150 lbs. or less. Drink 16 oz. if you weigh 151 pounds or more.

1 Lemon (slice it in wedges) One large bottle of Unfiltered Apple Juice

Morning
Drink the bottle of Olive Oil straight if possible. You can mix a little of the Unfiltered Apple Juice with it to help it get down but get the entire bottle down. Chase it by sucking on a lemon wedge if you feel like it's trying to "come back up". It should begin working within 24 hours or less.

During the cleanse and for 3 days eat live vegetables and fruits. NO SUGAR, PROCESSED FOODS, FRIED FOODS, FLOUR, MEATS, STARCHES, OR FATS. Drink unfiltered apple juice and distilled water only.

During the cleanse the oil will attach itself to excess sediment matter in the body, sludge build-up in the colon, kidneys, liver, gall bladder and spleen. You should actually see the gallstones pass through you. They will look like bright green peas. Most people have surgery to have those removed.

On day three you can begin introducing broth into your system. If you need meat, make sure it's grilled poultry or seafood only. However, you should try your best to eat as clean as possible from this point on so you don't defeat the purpose of the cleanse.

~CLEAN YOUR HOUSE AND EAT CLEAN~

In order to give yourself the best advantage at the beginning of this journey, I suggest that you go through your entire kitchen and discard, donate or give away the fattening, foods, foods that are high in caloric intake, fat, carbs, sodium, and sugar. This will require that you become a label reader and become educated on foods. Guard yourself from any foods that you know you struggle to resist because they are overly tempting to you.

Become a clean eater by eating healthy "live plant-based foods". Live foods are foods that are uncooked, unprocessed, wild, organic foods that consist of raw fruits, vegetables, nuts, seeds, eggs, fish, meat, and non-pasteurized/non-homogenized dairy products. Meats should be prepared as grilled, baked, or broiled. Buy organic if at all possible and avoid all genetically modified foods. Avoid all fried foods, candy and all processed sugary foods and drinks.

~IT DOESN'T COST AS MUCH AS YOU THINK TO EAT HEALTHY~

Many people believe that it has to cost a small fortune in order to eat healthy and well-balanced diet and that's totally untrue. There are many ways to shop smart. It may take a little work and planning on your part but it can be done. A few ways you can maximize your dollars and eat healthy are by:

- Planting a vegetable garden

- Shopping at Farmer's Markets

- Families partner together and purchase in Bulk at the Club stores and divide the items in half

- Freeze Leftovers

- Coupons

~TAKE BEFORE AND AFTER PHOTOS OF YOUR PROGRESS~

Take a photo of yourself on the first day of your lifestyle change. Continue to take photographs of yourself each month and post them in visible places like your mirror, refrigerator, or cabinets. Doing so serves as a great motivation tool and a deterrent to eating something unhealthy.

Purchase an item of clothing that is the size you desire to achieve and hang in a visible part of your house so you can see it daily.

~MAKE YOURSELF A PRIORITY~

If you're new to this, the type that's used to placing yourself on the back-burner or prone to make excuses, you will need to make yourself a priority by scheduling and making time for it and let nothing except an emergency get in your way.

There may be times when you will need to modify your workout routine but you must be determined and make yourself a priority and see putting yourself first and it as a form of guilt-free self-love. This is even if it takes you away from your family for an hour or two, this form of "me-time" is necessary for you to be your absolute best for you and your family. It's an absolute must.

~JUST GET MOVING~

The first time I walked back into a gym was over eight years ago. The gym was located in the apartment complex where I resided. I walked in and began walking on the treadmill. I lasted only about fifteen minutes. I started off great, gained rhythm, momentum and enough confidence to let go of the side-rails, fell and skinned my knee. Boy I was embarrassed. I picked myself up along with my pride and left. I returned the next day.

One day led to another and the pounds began to come off. I continued this regimen until I moved out of the complex three years later. I purchased a Gym membership at a community gym and continued my workout regimen and continue to do so to this day. I exercise 5 to 7 days a week and I also own light equipment in my home and use it during extreme inclement weather days or days when the Gym is closed for maintenance.

~GIVE THE SCALES A BREAK~
(At least in the beginning)

I rarely weigh myself. This is because in my younger years, I used to get on the bathroom scale over 10 times a day. It truly became an obsession. Today, I only weigh myself a few times a year. I gauge my progress by my clothes, pictures and how I look in the mirror. I encourage you in the beginning to give the scales a break because in the beginning of journey, you may gain weight due to muscle gain and inches lost. Always remember that muscle weighs more than fat.

~CELEBRATE YOUR NON-SCALE VICTORIES~

Always celebrate you non-scale victories!

Some non-scale victories come in the form of:

- Looser clothing

- Inches lost

- Smaller Clothes/Shoe Size

- Feeling better

~*Part 6*~

SETBACKS AND

SIDE~EFFECTS

~PLATEAUS~

There are times when you may experience a plateau in your health and wellness journey. A plateau is common especially with women that desire to lose a lot of weight. Don't allow this kind of setback to discourage you. Over time, our bodies get used to what we do physically on a consistent basis. We must constantly "trick our bodies" by modifying our workout and diet regimens. Consider modifying your workout routine every 4-6 weeks and increase your cardio time. Modify your carbohydrate sources every 4-6 weeks also. Eventually, your plateau should break on its own.

~EXCESS SKIN~

Sagging skin is one the side-effects of my weight-loss success. Sometimes women can experience sagging of the skin in various areas when losing weight. This is very common with women that have had bariatric (weight-loss) surgery. I suggest that you lift weights through the process and take runs and powerwalks if possible. I've never seen a runner with a large mid-section.

~AVOID TOXIC UNHEALTHY RELATIONSHIPS~

I know what it's like to experience unhealthy relationships with the opposite sex. I am have several and experienced abuse and its affects.

I'm a living testimony that you can overcome abuse on every level (emotional, psychological and physical) by going through the steps to heal, forgive, and become whole.

Many years ago and after I reached my goal weight, I met a man and had an exclusive relationship with him. Unfortunately, his eating habits were the total opposite of mine. He was not physically fit nor did he exercise.

In the beginning I attempted to use my power of influence to encourage him to work out with me as a guest at my Gym and would attempt to encourage him to eat healthier. He worked out with me only about three times and was only receptive to eating healthy once a week or so.

Over a two year period, I allowed his eating habits to influence me and my eating habits changed. I also was not consistent with my workout regimen because of the time I was investing in the relationship. This relationship ended abruptly and when it did, I was about twenty five pounds heavier than my goal weight.

I accepted responsibility for allowing myself to be influenced by those poor examples, immediately returned back to my original health and wellness regimen and lost the additional weight in a few months!

Yes! I still remember when I went in the closet to try on a pair of jeans that I once couldn't fit and the feeling when I was able to fit them! I shouted for joy! I made a vow to myself to never date another man that I wasn't equally yoked with when it came to diet and exercise.

~WEIGHT-LOSS SURGERY~

Many people that knew me at my heavier weight automatically assumed that I had some sort of bariatric weight-loss surgery. In the beginning it felt like a compliment but I will admit over time, I began to find it somewhat irritating. When you know that you worked hard to get healthy, the comments and assumptions of taking what I'll call, "a more convenient" way out can become a bit much.

I have often been asked what my views are concerning bariatric surgery. I don't put down anyone that makes surgery their method of choice and support them. All I say when asked is that whatever the route you choose to lose weight must be MANAGED. I know a few women that chose this route and have gained the weight they lost back.

The body is very forgiving to the point that the skin's elasticity is forgiving both ways.

~NO SECRETS OR MAGIC TRICKS~

Many people in my home state of California became aware of my drastic weight loss via online Social Media. I remember about six and a half years ago having a three way phone conversation with two women from my home state that were absolutely amazed at how much weight I loss. The first thing they asked me was "what's your secret"? I was on the phone for almost 3 hours trying to answer their questions. I told them exactly what I did and it was like they didn't believe me. They continued to ask me the same repetitive questions in different ways. I remained polite and kept giving them the same answers but after 2 hours, I was beginning to feel as if I were on a witness stand undergoing interrogation (laughing out loud)! I ended the call by telling them that there's no secret or magic trick. It must be a lifestyle change. Just begin by praying, making slow gradual changes in your diet, incorporate exercise and consistency and you will see results.

~THE YO'YO SYNDROME~

I experienced fluctuations in my weight loss about 3 times in my younger years. Those times was I was uneducated, and didn't see it as a lifestyle change. I was totally ignorant thinking that after losing the weight that I could return to my former eating habits. I couldn't have been more WRONG.

It is very important to be consistent as possible in maintaining your goal weight once you achieve it. Yo'Yo'ing up and down affects the body's metabolism and can work against you in the long run.

IT'S A LIFESTYLE CHANGE.

~MAINTAINING AND KEEPING THE WEIGHT OFF~

I have lost a total of over one hundred forty pounds from my heaviest lifetime weight to my lightest weight nine+ years ago. Now, that's a whole person plus a few pounds.

Due to hormones, my weight has fluctuates sometimes from five to ten pounds. However, I am happy to say that I have successfully kept over one hundred plus pounds off for over the last nine plus years and counting. I don't weigh myself as often as most. I self-monitor my progress by my clothes size, photographs and how I look and it works for me.

~*Part 7*~

AUDRA'S ORIGINAL
MEAL PLAN

~MY ORIGINAL MEAL PLAN~

Below is the original meal plan that I created and designed on my own and used to "jump start" my health and wellness journey.

I have categorized them under Breakfast, Lunch, & Dinner. I pick and choose 1 or 2 from each category. Just do what works for you. This is not a specific diet. I just sort of experimented with it, and developed the plan as I went along, and saw progress. The main things I pay attention to are: Carbs, Sodium, Fat, Saturated Fat, Sugar, Fiber, and Protein. You must become a label reader if you want to be successful in this journey.

BREAKFAST (Drink at least 1 small bottle 16.9 FL oz. of water before eating)

Quaker Oatmeal or Special K (Protein Plus) Cereal

(Cereal Box is Light Blue in the front)

1/4 or 1/2 Grapefruit or 1/2 of an Orange

SNACK (Between 10:00 & 11:00 a.m. and 2:00 & 3:00 p.m.)

(Drink at least 1 small bottle 16.9 oz. of water before eating)

1/4 or 1/2 can of Fruit Cocktail or Sliced Peaches w/Splenda (No Sugar Added)

Or other 1/2 of the Orange or Grapefruit

Cottage Cheese w/fruit

Quaker Reduced Sugar Granola Bar (90 Calories)

Sugar Free Jell-O

LUNCH (Drink at least 1 small bottle 16.9 FL oz. of water before eating)

Salad with or without Grilled Chicken (with Reduced Fat Dressing)

Campbell's "Healthy Request" Soups (Savory Chicken & Rice, Chicken & Pasta or Mexican Tortilla)

These soups have 40% to 50% less sodium than the regular soups & can range from 110 to 190 calories per can

Reduced Fat Crackers

DINNER (Drink at least 1 small bottle 16.9 FL oz. of water before eating)

I basically alternate from the Lunch Menu most of

the time (e.g. Soup for Lunch, Salad for Dinner or

vice versa). However, I do sometimes eat the

following to give myself a break:

Chicken Breast or Ground Turkey Patty grilled on the George Foreman Grill

Frozen Peas or Corn or Broccoli (Frozen or Fresh)

Frozen veggies carry less Sodium than canned ones

1/2 baked Potato

DESSERT OR SNACK AFTER DINNER

100 Calorie Pack Chips a' Hoy or

Sugar Free Jell-O & Fruit Cocktail w/Fat Free or Sugar Free Cool Whip

BEVERAGES OTHER THAN WATER

Non-Carbonated Beverages (Look for the

Low Carb varieties) these drinks are very low

calorie and are infused with vitamins & minerals.

Diet Green Tea

Sugar Free infused Beverages

Fruit Infused Water

SWEETENERS: Splenda or Stevia

I also drink ORGANIC APPLE CIDER VINEGAR in my water 2-3 times daily. The vinegar has many benefits. Just make sure that the vinegar you purchase has what is called, "THE MOTHER" in it. The Mother is the sediment that settles at the bottom of the bottle.

FOODS TO AVOID

Fried Foods, Starches, Breads, Candy, foods with refined sugars or anything rich or that you know is a "food taboo" for you. Don't even keep junk food in the house for guests if you can help it.

SUPPLEMENTS

Take your vitamin supplements, and drink plenty of Water throughout the day. I drink about 1 and 1/2 gallons daily.

Consider adding Whey Protein to your supplement regimen after each workout, within thirty minutes is the optimal time for protein synthesis, but is not mandatory. Consult with your Physician before starting any supplement regimen.

EXERCISE REGIMEN

Try to work out from 30 to 60 minutes 1-2 times a day. If you're unable to get to the gym, exercising in your home can be as just as effective. Walking is really good. Make sure that you incorporate Cardio in your workout daily because Cardio serves as the "fat burner". Use the weights to develop muscle tone and reduce as well.

Exercise in the bathroom stall each time you use the restroom while at work by doing a couple of sets of squats or wall pushups. Studies show that women in our age group will lose 1/2 pound of muscle every year during our adult life but can increase our strength 100% in just 12 weeks. Our bodies get used to what we do so remember: PUSH YOURSELF AND CHANGE UP YOUR WORKOUT PERIODICALLY TO BREAK ANY PLATEAUS.

~AFFIRMATIONS~

Write a list of positive affirmations of what you want to see happen to your body and the reasons why you want to lose weight on a Post-It and place it on your bathroom mirror and read aloud daily.

~STRESS EATING~

It's easy to resort to junk food when stressed because it is faster to soothe us when we encounter stressful situations. We know that stress is just a part of life and that stress does affect our emotions. Eating out of emotions is not good but if you must have something, to eat, make sure that it' something healthy like a fruit or vegetable. Before you put it in your mouth, stop, think and ask yourself, why am I eating or why do I want to eat. If you know that it is from a stressor then try your best doing something other than eating. Consider releasing the stress by writing down how you're feeling.

~MAKE IT A FAMILY AFFAIR~

I want to encourage you to make it a family affair! My son joined me in his own personal journey last year and he has made great strides and looks phenomenal!

~PERSONAL HEALING TESTIMONY~

In late 2010, I had an abnormal mammogram. Tests revealed 2 nodules/cysts in one breast. My Physician told me that he wanted to keep a close watch on them required that I report to have ultrasounds every 6 months. I did as told and reported to the Dr.'s office for ultrasounds every 6 months for 2 ½ years while praying and speaking positive affirmations of life and health in my breasts and death to those nodules/cyst by commanding them be eradicated in Jesus name.

In the fall of 2013, I returned to the Dr'. office and for an ultrasound and the technician was amazed. He kept prodding around looking for those nodules/cysts and couldn't find them. He left and got the Doctor and the doctor prodded around with the ultrasound instrument. The Doctor and technician excused themselves for a moment.

They returned about 5 minutes later and said that they didn't see any evidence nodules/cysts and that 6 month screenings were no longer necessary!

This is a testimony to how forgiving the body is to itself even if your have to walk it out with prayer, unwavering faith and a proper diet.

I believe that the body is always looking for ways to compensate and heal itself to the best of its ability. Just like when a person skins their knee, immediately after the body begins to activate what's necessary to begin the healing process.

In closing, I would like to encourage you to by saying that it's never too late to start. If you fall short today, you will have 24 hours given to you the next. You can start over anytime.

I could do it, anyone can. Please let me know how you're doing. It is my prayer that God will keep us all health conscious and mindful of what we put into our bodies because our body is the "Temple of the Holy Spirit". **ENJOY THE JOURNEY!**

ACKNOWLEDGEMENTS

First and foremost, I would like to give thanks to God for making all things possible for me. Second, I am thankful to my amazing family, my parents, John and Mary for their love, upbringing, and guidance. My children Brandon and Lisa for their own personal success and joining me and in their own health and wellness journey.

I am especially thankful for the late Federico "Rico" Brown who served as my Online Fitness motivator and Coach. Pastors James H. Davis and Pastor Otha Turnbough for sowing and contributing greatly to my spiritual growth.

Dr. Cindy Trimm for a teaching that changed my life.

My spiritual sisters and prayer partners Janeese, Pauline, Dominique, Candance, Shay &

Lisa. These Women of God have always encouraged me and prayed me through.

Author Keith Murphy helped me resurrect my passion for writing that laid dormant for many, many years.

Edward Jordan who inspired me behind the scenes to cross the finish line. My Doctor for gently prodding me to take action and responsibility. My Facebook Sisters in the group, "Sister's Getting Fit for the Kingdom."

DISCLAIMER: Audra Johnson is not a licensed physician, dietician or psychologist. She does not guarantee that readers will receive the same results as she did.

This book is personal her testimony of what worked for her and realizes that results may vary. She does not assume or guarantee responsibility for the outcomes experienced by readers.

Please consult your physician before starting this or any other diet, fitness or supplement regimen.

AUDRA'S PHOTOS

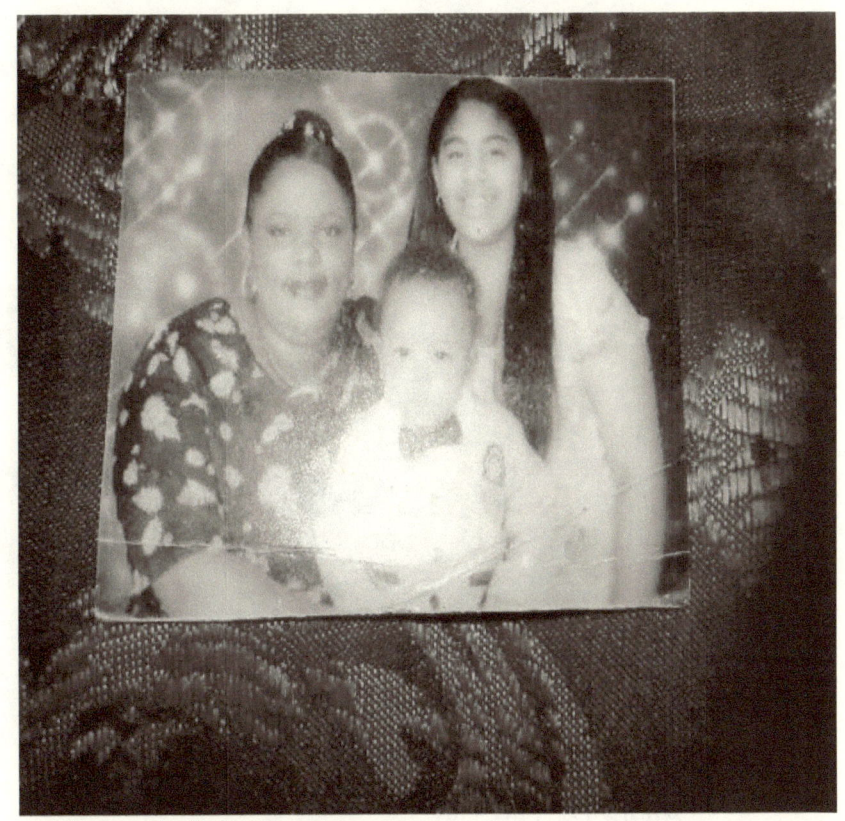

Audra on the left 18 years ago.

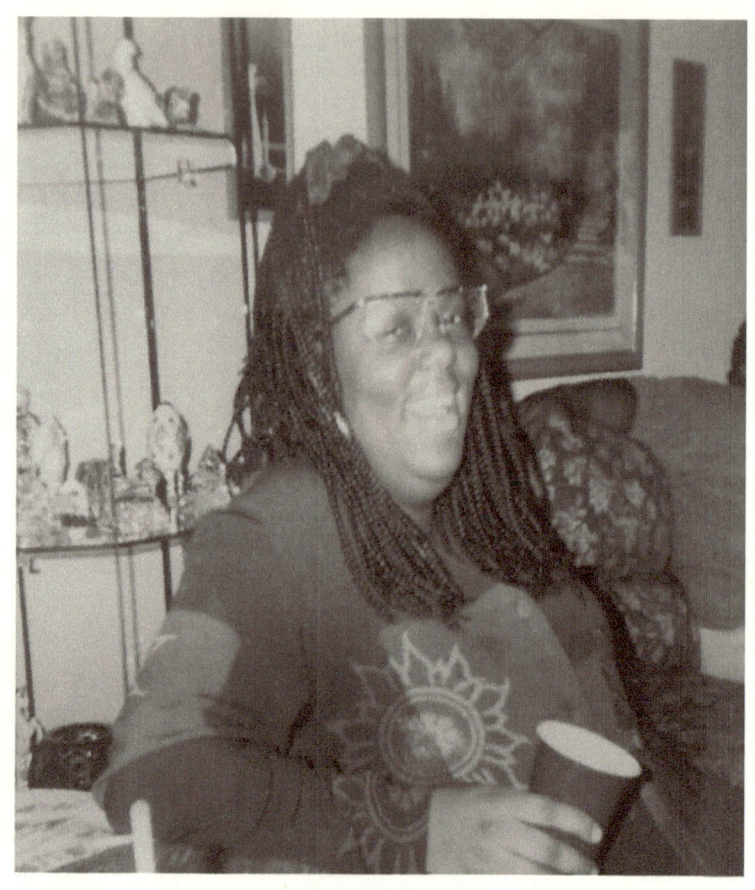

Audra 18 years ago

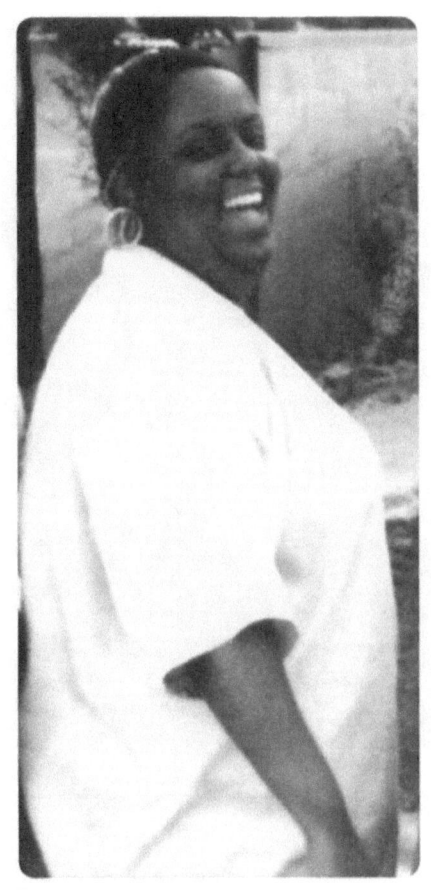 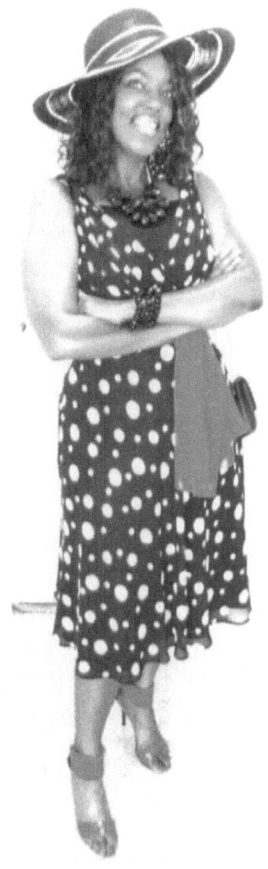

Audra 19 years ago   Audra 2015

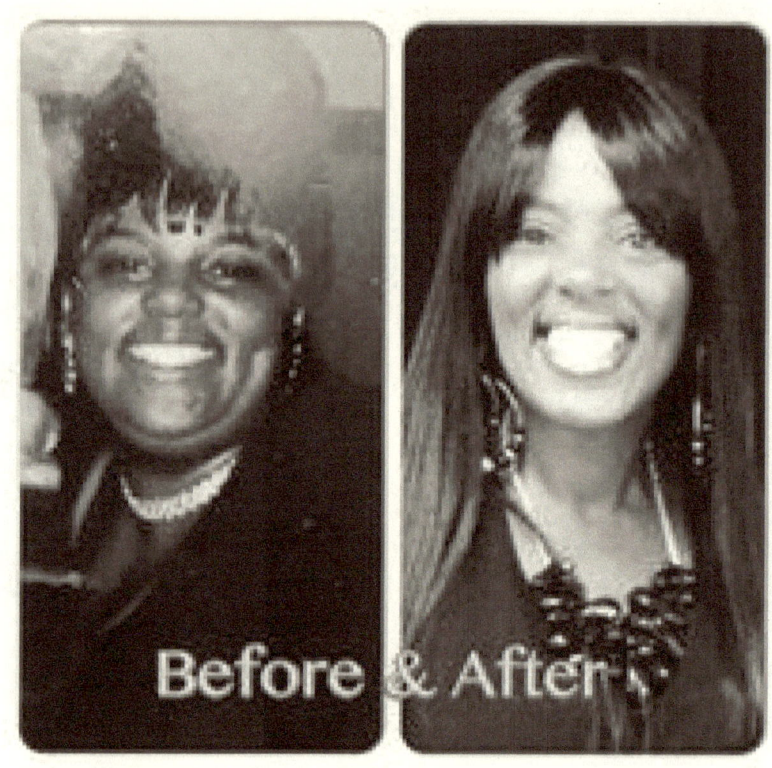

Audra Before   Audra After

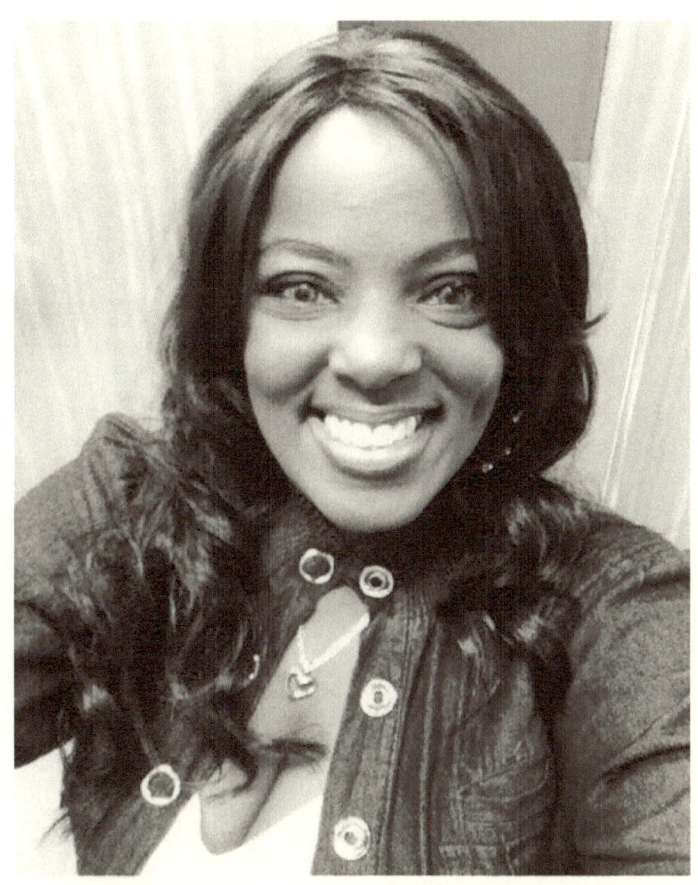

Audra After

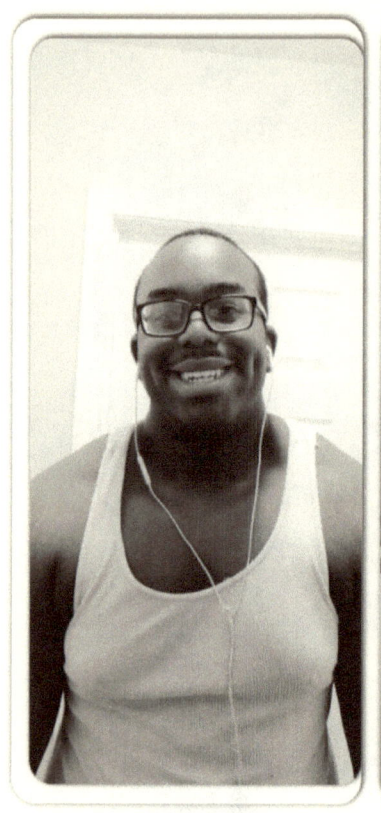 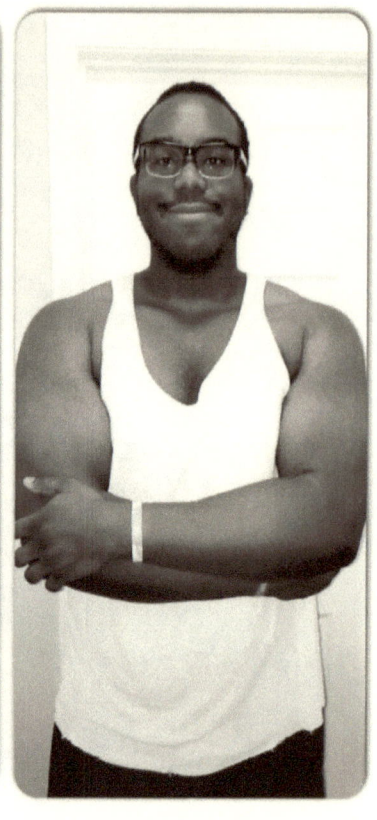

My Son 2014   My Son 2015

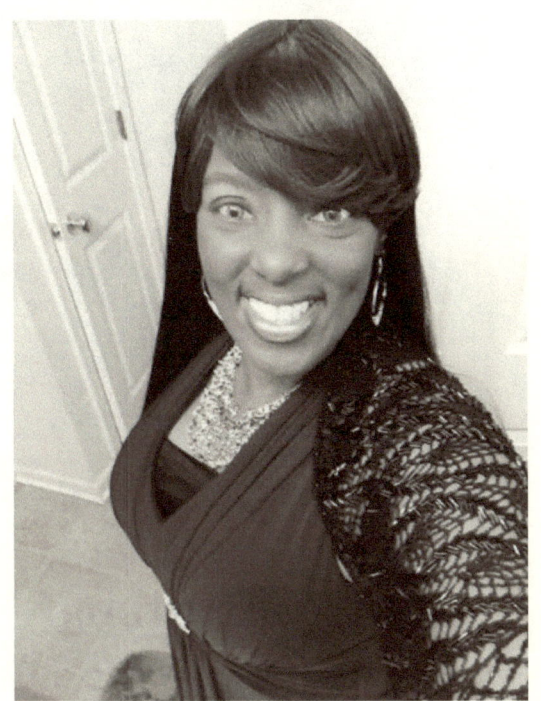

Audra in 2015 wearing a size 6 dress

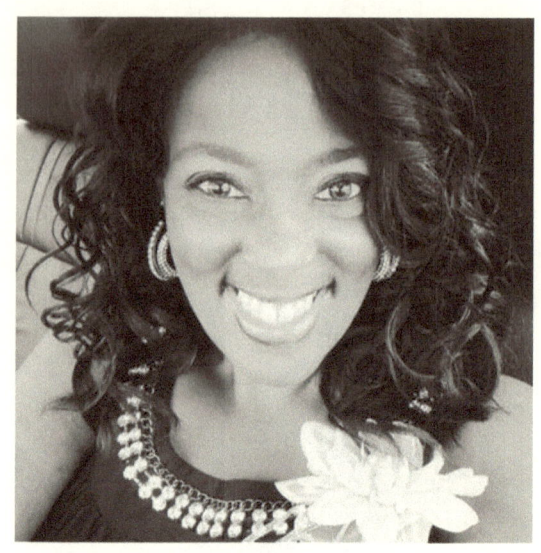

ABOUT THE AUTHOR

Audra is a Single-Parent, Minister and founder of Living Victorious Ministries and serves in many facets of Ministry. She attends Eternal Life Harvest Center Church in Knoxville, TN.

One of her callings and assignments is to help restore the broken and abused Sisterhood. Her passion is to help people overcome obesity by making slow, gradual changes in their diet and fitness regimen.

Her testimonies have been featured on Health and Wellness Websites such as:

- Black Women Losing Weight

- Not Really Hungry

- Black Women Do Workout

She is also a writer, poet, motivational speaker and founder of the Facebook group, Sister's Getting Fit For The Kingdom. She started this group as a source of encouragement source to those that have reached their health and wellness goals and those that desire to lose weight and live healthier lives. The link to access the group page is: https://www.facebook.com/groups/3826477050884 58/

She is available for speaking engagements and/or conferences of all kinds and can be

reached at: livingvictorious14@yahoo.com and

on Instagram at: @livingvictorious1

BODY
FORGIVENESS

www.ingramcontent.com/pod-product-compliance
Lightning Source LLC
Chambersburg PA
CBHW050428290526
45786CB00003B/1443